1

TABLE OF CONTENTS

INTRODUCTION

Cayenne pepper has been prized for thousands of years for its healing power. Folklore from around the world recounts amazing results using cayenne pepper in simple healing and in baffling health problems. But cayenne pepper is not just a healer from ancient history. Recent clinical studies have been conducted on many of the old-time health applications for this miracle herb. Again and again, the therapeutic value of cayenne pepper has been medically validated.

Many herbalists believe that Cayenne is the most useful and valuable herb in the herb kingdom, not only for the entire digestive system, but also for the heart and circulatory system. It acts as a catalyst and increases the effectiveness of other herbs when used with them. Cayenne is a medicinal and nutritional herb. It is a very high source of Vitamins A and C, has the complete B complexes, and is very rich in organic calcium and potassium, which is one of the reasons it is good for the heart.

Cayenne can rebuild the tissue in the stomach and the peristaltic action in the intestines. It aids elimination and assimilation, and helps the body to create hydrochloric acid, which is so necessary for good digestion and assimilation, especially of proteins. All this becomes very significant when we realize that the digestive system plays the most important role in mental, emotional and physical health, as it is through the digestive system that the brain, glands, muscles and every other part of the body are fed.

Cayenne has been known to stop heart attacks within 30 seconds. For example, when a 90-year-old man in Oregon had a severe heart attack, his daughter was able to get Cayenne extract into his mouth. He was pronounced dead by the medics, but within a few minutes, he regained consciousness. On the way to the hospital, he remained in a semi-conscious state, but the daughter kept giving him the Cayenne extract. By the time they got to the hospital, he had fully recovered and wanted to go home and mow the lawn. The doctor asked what she had given him, as he said it was the closest thing to a miracle he had ever seen.

Cayenne pepper is said to be unequal for its ability to boost circulation and increase heart action. Capsicum exerts a variety of desirable actions on the entire cardiovascular system. It has the extraordinary ability to enhance cardiovascular performance while actually lowering blood pressure. Capsicum has an energizing effect on the entire system. It has traditionally been used for overcoming fatigue and restoring stamina and vigor. It is a natural stimulant without the threatening side effects (palpitations, hyper-activity or rise in blood pressure) of most other stimulating agents.

CAYENNE PEPPER

Cayenne is a shrub that originated in Central and South America and now grows in subtropical and tropical climates. Its hollow fruit grows into long pods that turn red, orange or yellow when they ripen.

Cayenne chili peppers (or Capsicum frutescens) belong to the genus Capsicum and come from a similar cultivar of Capsicum annuum. Capsicum is an herb, and the fruit of the capsicum plant is used to make medicine.

The cayenne pepper is a thin chili pepper, green to red in color, about 2 to 5 inches long. The "cayenne pepper" spice you use mostly in pizza restaurants is the dried, ground version of this pepper.

It belongs to the nightshade family of flowering plants and are related to bell peppers and jalapenos.

The word cayenne comes from the city of Cayenne in French Guiana. Cayenne is great in soups and sauces, on pizzas, as well as over meats and seafoods. Keep it on the table in a shaker as an alternative to salt or pepper.

Cayenne pepper is typically added to food in either its natural or powdered form, and some people use it as a cream or capsule in order to take advantage of its detoxifying properties.

Cayenne pepper benefits are numerous. It's used to help digestion, including heal upset stomach, slow intestinal gas, stop stomach pain, stop diarrhea and as a natural remedy for cramps.

It's also used for conditions of the heart and blood vessels — including to improve poor circulation, reverse excessive blood clotting, lower high cholesterol and prevent heart disease.

When consumed, cayenne pepper has the power to relieve a toothache, seasickness, alcoholism, malaria and fever. It's also used to help people who have difficulty swallowing.

When applied topically, cayenne pepper benefits the skin, too.

Currently, it's being studied to test its ability to reduce pain sensations when applied to the skin, and research indicates that it would be effective as a remedy for headaches (including migraines), potential solution for osteoarthritis and other painful conditions.

Many of these cayenne pepper benefits are possible because of the plant's active compound capsaicin. This molecule works by binding to a vanilloid receptor known as TRPV1, which triggers a mild inflammatory reaction that's meant to repair injured cells.

disease, rheumatism, and even the common cold, along with many other health problems.

• Cayenne Buist's Yellow Chili Pepper

The Cayenne Buist's Yellow is an excellent salsa pepper, and works well dehydrated and crushed into powder for various seasoning applications.

The Cayenne Buist's chili pepper originated in the United States. The pods are a bright orange and grow to roughly 4-5 inches in length. The pepper plant is quite productive, producing a lot of fruit which start out green and ripen to a gorgeous golden orange. The pods are somewhat sweet and rather mild in heat level.

• Dagger Pod Chili Peppers – Cayenne Type

The "Dagger Pod" is a hot cayenne chili pepper that grows to 4-5 inches long by ½ to ¾ inches wide. It is a long, thin, and pointy, somewhat resembling a dagger – pendant shaped.

It is a thin fleshed pepper that starts off green and matures to a vibrant red.

It is a mid season pepper, producing pods in 70-80 days.

It is a very prolific plant producing many, many pods.

Use the dagger pod as you would use any cayenne chili pepper. It is usedfor making hot sauces or for drying and grinding into vibrant powders and seasoning blends.

• Cayenne Golden Chili Peppers

The very attractive Golden Cayenne matures from green to a beautiful golden yellow with smoother skin and fewer wrinkles than the traditional red cayenne pepper. They also grow a bit larger than the red cayenne, about 4-6 inches long, but with the same slim, tapered, and slightly twisted shape.

Since their heat develops as they grow larger, wait until maturity to harvest in order to get the full heat. Use the Golden Cayenne in just about any dish in which you might use a jalapeno or habanero, but be ready for significantly more heat than a jalapeno.

Specifically, Golden Cayennes are fantastic when used in Creole, Cajun and Southern cooking. Like most hot peppers, they can be roasted and used in salsa, hot sauces and jellies.

They also dry nicely and can be ground into a very attractive golden chili powder. Perhaps the best feature of these peppers is their attractive shape and color which add variety and beauty to your garden.

How to Grow Cayenne Pepper Plants

Growing cayenne pepper plants requires some heat. Chilies are mostly perennial in their native habitat of sub-tropical and tropical regions. If you live in an area that has a long growing season and a lot of sun, you may directly sow seeds in the garden 10-14 days before the last frost date.

In temperate areas, chilies are grown as annuals, so when starting cayenne pepper plants from seed, it's best to do so indoors or in a greenhouse. They are very delicate and react badly to overly hot or cold weather. Sow the seeds in light, well-drained soil medium and keep in a sunny location at a temperature of at least 60 F. (16 C.) until the seeds sprout in 16-20 days.

Plant the growing cayenne pepper seedlings into flats spaced 2-3 inches apart or in individual pots and allow to gradually acclimate or harden to outdoor temperatures. Generally, outdoor transplanting should occur six to eight weeks after the seeds are sown, or after all danger of frost has passed; however, if you choose to transplant before the weather is frost free, it is advisable to protect the plants with row covers, hot caps and/or transplant the peppers through black plastic.

To prepare for transplanting the cayenne pepper plants, amend the soil with fertilizer or organic compound, if need be, avoiding too much nitrogen in an area of full sun to mostly full exposure. Plant your pepper babies 18-24 inches (46 to 61 cm.) apart in a row.

Care of Cayenne Peppers

Moist soil is required in the care of cayenne peppers but take care not to overwater. Saturated soil, or overly dry soil for that matter, may cause the foliage to yellow. Organic mulch or plastic sheeting help reduce weeding and conserve water; however, do not apply organic mulch until the soil has warmed to 75 F. (24 C.). Cayenne pepper plants may overwinter if protected from frost or moved inside. Prune the plants as needed.

Cayenne peppers will be ready to harvest in about 70-80 days. When ready, cayenne pepper will be 4-6 inches (10 to 15 cm.) long and easily pull from the stem, although it is really better to snip from the plant so you do not cause any damage. Some fruit will be green, partially green or colored and should be stored at a temperature of 55 F. (13 C.). Harvesting will be ongoing and continue until the first frost of fall.

HERBAL STIMULANT

When you hear the word stimulant it is easy for thoughts of caffeine or methamphetamines to come to mind. These drug-like constituents are indeed stimulants.

But in the herbal world stimulants have a broader, more energetic meaning. Simply defined, a stimulant is something that increases the energy output of a system or organ.

Caffeine and meth are nervous system stimulants. They increase the energy output of the nervous system, leaving the consumer feeling hyped-up or wired.

Exercise can be thought of as a stimulant too. Rapid movement increases the energy output of the cardiovascular system, respiratory system, nervous system, etc.

Cayenne is also a stimulant. It specifically effects the cardiovascular system, mucous membranes and digestion.

Nutrition Facts of Cayenne Pepper.

Cayenne pepper contains vitamin C, vitamin B6, vitamin E, potassium, manganese and flavonoids – which provide its powerful antioxidant properties.

On the Scoville Rating Scale, cayenne pepper is rated typically anywhere from 30,000 to 190,000 Scoville Heat Units (SHU). (Pure capsaicin has the highest SHU rating.)

Here are the cayenne pepper nutrition facts, listed in recommended daily values. One teaspoon (about two grams) of cayenne pepper contains approximately:

• 5.6 calories

• 1 gram carbohydrates

• 0.2 grams protein

- 0.3 grams fat

- 0.5 grams fiber

- 728 international units vitamin A (15 percent DV)

- 0.5 milligrams vitamin E (3 percent DV)

- 1.3 milligrams vitamin C (2 percent DV)

- 1.4 micrograms vitamin K (2 percent DV)

Health Benefits of Cayenne pepper

1. Helps Digestion

One of the major cayenne pepper benefits is the positive effect it has on the digestive system.

Cayenne pepper helps produce saliva, which is important for excellent digestion as well as preventing bad breath. Research suggests that consuming cayenne pepper stimulates our salivary glands, which is needed to begin the digestive process.

Cayenne pepper also stimulates the flow of enzyme production, which is essential for our digestive system to work properly. It also stimulates gastric juices that aid the body's ability to metabolize food and toxins.

2. Relieves Migraine Pain

Researchers suggest that cayenne pepper, due to its spice, is able to stimulate a pain response in a different part of the body. Once this happens, the brain puts its attention on that new site and will no longer concentrate on the pain in the head, which causes the migraine headache.

After this initial pain reaction from the cayenne pepper, the nerve fibers have a depleted substance P, or pain chemical, and the sensation of pain is lessened.

With cayenne compounds, you're basically tricking your body to "feel pain" somewhere else, so that the head is no longer the main focus for pain chemicals.

3. Prevents Blood Clots

Blood clots are blockages in your arteries and blood vessels that limit blood flow through your circulatory system.

Cayenne encourages fibrinolytic activity and helps prevent blood clots. This is also the reason why cayenne pepper is effective in preventing heart attacks.

Studies indicate that the capsaicin in cayenne pepper helps to clear away artery-narrowing lipid deposits, and dilates arteries and blood vessels to clear away clots.

4. Provides Detox Support

Cayenne pepper benefits include its ability to stimulate circulation and eliminate acidity.

According to research published in Critical Reviews in Food Science and Nutrition, cayenne pepper restores the circulatory system by opening the capillaries and regulating blood sugar; it also helps the digestive system that moves bacteria and toxins out of the body.

Research conducted in the Netherlands suggests that cayenne pepper also increases body temperature and boosts your metabolism.

5. Relieves Joint and Nerve Pain

Cayenne power has very powerful pain-relieving properties when applied to the skin. It reduces the amount of substance P, a chemical that carries pain messages to the brain. When there is less substance P, the pain messages no longer reach the brain and you feel relief.

Studies have found that cayenne pepper relieves pain after surgery, such as a mastectomy or an amputation.

It also alleviates pain from nerve damage in the feet or legs from diabetes, lower back injuries, neuropathy, osteoarthritis and rheumatoid arthritis, as well as fibromyalgia symptoms like joint or muscle pain.

6. Supports Weight Loss

A study published in PloS One found that consuming cayenne pepper for breakfast creates less appetite, so people eat less calories during the day.

It also burns excess fat because it's a metabolic booster. As one of the key anti-inflammatory foods, cayenne pepper benefits also include weight loss.

Cayenne pepper has the power to soothe inflammation and bloating that comes from allergies, food sensitivities and infections.

7. Works as Anti-Irritant

Cayenne pepper benefits include its anti-irritant properties, making it effective in easing ulcers, upset stomachs, cough and even potentially stop diarrhea.

The common belief is that cayenne pepper, when consumed in excessive amounts, leads to gastric ulcers because of its irritant and acid-secreting nature.

People with ulcers are actually advised to limit or avoid using cayenne pepper; however, investigations carried out in recent years have revealed that chili, or its active principle "capsaicin," is not the cause for the formation of ulcer symptoms but a benefactor.

Studies have found that cayenne pepper does not stimulate, but inhibits acid secretion, stimulates alkali and mucus secretions and particularly gastric mucosal blood flow, which helps in the prevention and healing of ulcers.

8. Treats Psoriasis

Psoriasis occurs when skin cells replicate too quickly, and it results in swollen patches under the skin covered with whitish scales on top. The scaly patches are areas of inflammation and excessive skin production.

Two trials showed that 0.025 percent capsaicin (cayenne pepper) cream used topically is effective in treating psoriasis.

The first study showed a significant decrease in scaling and redness during a six-week period in 44 patients with moderate and severe psoriasis.

The second was a double-blind study of 197 patients, which found that psoriasis was treated with the capsaicin cream four times daily for six weeks, with a significant decrease in scaling, thickness, redness and itching.

9. Boosts Metabolism

Cayenne pepper benefits also include its ability to regulate your metabolism, according to a review published in Open Heart.

It has been found to effectively suppress hunger and normalize glucose levels. It also keeps blood pressure levels normalized, and helps the body lower LDL cholesterol and triglycerides.

People with cold and stagnant digestion have a difficult time transforming food into nutrients. They are often experiencing fatigue due to the exhaustive energy being used to attempt digestion. They are further disadvantaged because their poor digestion leaves them lacking the nutrients needed to feel vibrant.

Symptoms of stagnant and cold digestion include:

- Bloating

- Belching

- Sour regurgitation

- Nausea

- Foul breath

- Gas

- Lack of appetite

- Loose stools

- Undigested food in stools

- Heartburn

- Feeling of coldness in the limbs or in the stomach

- Tongue is swollen, wet, with possible heavy white coating

- Abdominal pain that is relieved with pressure

Cayenne is a premier herb for warming and stimulating digestion. It can be added to foods, taken as tea or a capsule (careful not to take too much!) or used in a tincture.

10. Fights Cold and Flu

Cayenne pepper benefits include being full of beta carotene and antioxidants that support your immune system.

It aids in breaking up and moving congested mucus, and once this nasty mucus leaves the body, the symptoms of the flu or cold will diminish.

Besides helping as a natural remedy for the flu, cayenne pepper also raises your body temperature, which makes you sweat and increases the activity of your immune system. As a vitamin C food, cayenne pepper may also help you to kick that nasty cold.

Cayenne peppers can help prevent a cold or flu as well as shorten the duration of a cold or flu. They bring heat to the body, which can help to dispel coldness (in Traditional Chinese Medicine some colds and the flu are brought on by a cold invasion). Sweating therapies, using saunas or hot baths as well as internal medicines like cayenne are a long-celebrated way to stop a cold in its tracks.

Cayenne also promotes secretions from the mucous membranes. Mucus is loaded with antibodies and is a powerful immune system response to an invading pathogen. If the cold or the flu has progressed and the person has stuffed up sinuses, cayenne peppers will quickly drain them! Moving congested mucus lessens the possibility of a secondary infection in the sinuses.

Cayenne peppers are high in Vitamin A, which is essential to mucus membrane health. Your mucus membranes are an important part of your immune system and keeping them healthy helps to prevent infections.

11. Source of Vitamin A

Vitamin A plays a critical role in maintaining healthy vision, neurological function and healthy skin; it is an antioxidant that reduces inflammation by fighting free radicals.

Studies have repeatedly shown that antioxidants like vitamin A are vital to good health and longevity; they benefit eye health, boost immunity and foster cell growth.

Lucky for us, cayenne pepper is a great source of vitamin A; in fact, with just two teaspoons of cayenne pepper, you are getting your fill of vitamin A for the day!

12. Contains Vitamin E

Vitamin E benefits include helping many organs in the body function properly and is extremely useful in naturally slowing the aging process.

This important and beneficial vitamin has the power to balance cholesterol, fight free radicals, repair damaged skin, balance hormones, repair damaged skin and hair, improve vision and increase energy levels ... and cayenne pepper is an important provider of vitamin E.

13. Prevents Allergies

Because cayenne is an anti-inflammatory agent, it has the power to prevent allergies and the symptoms related to allergies. A food allergy, for example, is a measurable response to consuming a specific food.

Food allergies, or intolerances, can be caused by a condition known as leaky gut (intestinal permeability), when proteins and food particles pass through the gut and cause systemic body inflammation.

Leaky gut is like having the gates broken from your intestines to your bloodstream so that toxins, microbes and undigested food particles can now get through. When this happens, it causes inflammation throughout your body, leading to a variety of diseases.

14. Possible Anti-Cancer Agent

Studies suggest that capsaicin may have a role as a natural remedy for cancer, including in the management of prostate cancer.

One study conducted at University of California at Los Angeles School of Medicine found that this important ingredient in cayenne pepper is able to inhibit the growth of cancer cells and prevent the activation of new dangerous formations.

There is also data from California's Loma Linda University that suggests that cayenne pepper benefits include being effective in helping prevent lung cancer in smokers.

Cayenne pepper's high amounts of capsaicin serves as a substance that can stop the formation of tobacco induced tumors in the lung. Similar effects have also been found in liver tumors when they were exposed to cayenne pepper.

15. Anti-Fungal Properties

The final cayenne pepper benefit is its ability to kill fungus and prevent the formation of fungal pathogens. Cayenne pepper was investigated to determine its in vitro antifungal activity, and the results found that it was active against 16 different fungal strains, including Candida.

Candida is a fungus that aids with nutrient absorption and digestion, when in proper levels in the body. When it overproduces, however, the typical candida symptoms may appear.

This includes hormone imbalance, joint pain, digestive problems and a weak immune system.

How to Use of Cayenne pepper

Cayenne peppers are available year-round in supermarkets or health food stores. You can find them in fresh, dried or powdered form.

Because powdered cayenne pepper is sometimes a mix a poorer quality herbs, it's best to buy cayenne peppers fresh; however, if you are using dried or powered pepper, the health benefits are still awesome.

Just be sure to buy your powder from a trusted company. Go for powders that are authentic and branded products — there are even organic options.

In the store, look for raw, fresh chilies that have a brilliant red color and a healthy stem. Make sure there aren't any spots, mold or spoiled tips.

The pepper should look wholesome and firm. Once at home, store your peppers inside the refrigerator in a plastic bag; they will stay fresh for about a week.

Dry peppers are also available at the supermarket, especially health food stores. Dry peppers can be stored using airtight containers in a cool and dark place.

Dried cayenne peppers can be milled to powder using a hand mill.

Fresh cayenne chili peppers can be used to make spicy drinks, sauce, chutney or can even be used for pickling. Make sure you wash them well first — you want to use any dirt, sand or fungicides.

Here's a breakdown of some simple ways to use cayenne in your daily health regime:

• Add it to meals: Taking cayenne pepper that is dried or powdered, you can add to meals for a spicy (and healthy) kick. It can be added to meat, pasta, eggs, nuts and veggies — there are a ton of options. Start with a ½ teaspoon or so, and then work your way up. Remember that it adds heat and can be too much for people who are spice-sensitive.

• Drink it: If you want a quick fix that will help you to experience these amazing cayenne pepper benefits, an easy way to get it in your body is by taking a cayenne pepper drink by mixing the powder with water and lemon, which is similar to the drink consumed during the cayenne pepper diet, so it will give you the same detoxifying results.

• Take capsules: Cayenne capsules or capsaicin capsules are also available for purchase. When taking cayenne pills, read the label carefully for dosage instructions. It's best to start with a lower dose to monitor how your body reacts.

• Apply it topically: There are also creams that contain capsaicin, the main component of cayenne pepper, that can be found in most stores. These creams are used to treat skin infections, sore muscles and tension. By rubbing a small amount of cream on the affected area, you will feel the pain and irritation subside. If you are using a cream, make sure to read the directions carefully so that you don't use too much. Also, be sure to wash your hands after applying capsaicin cream because it can cause a burning sensation on your hands; try washing with vinegar and water for the best results.

Interesting Facts

The chili originated in Central and South America. It's named after the capital city of the French Guiana, Cayenne. From seeds found on the floors of caves that were ancient human dwellings and from ancient fossil feces, scientists have found that people were eating peppers as early as 7000 B.C.

Cayenne is one of the main foods of the Hunzas in Asia, along with apricots and their pits, millet and other simple foods. These people live to over a hundred years of age, which some say is because of their natural immune-boosting and anti-inflammatory foods that they consume daily.

Cayenne peppers were even growing in the Hawaiian Islands in as early as 1897; these smaller and more pungent fruits were called "Hawaiian Chili Peppers."

Today, you can find cayenne pepper all over the world, and it now has a reputation for its health benefits.

Risks, Side Effects and Interactions

Medicinal lotions and creams that contain capsicum extract are known to be safe for most adults when applied to the skin and consumed. The active chemical in capsicum, capsaicin, is approved by the FDA as an over-the-counter product, so it can be sold without a prescription.

When applied topically, cayenne pepper side effects may include skin irritation, burning and itching. It can also be extremely irritating to the eyes, nose and throat, so be careful when using cayenne pepper on sensitive skin or around the eyes.

When consumed in moderate doses, side effects can include upset stomach and irritation, sweating, flushing and runny nose.

Because cayenne pepper may increase bleeding during and after surgery, it's best to stop using cayenne pepper as a natural medication at least two weeks before a scheduled surgery.

Medications that slow blood clotting, such as anticoagulant and antiplatelet drugs, interact with cayenne pepper and should be avoided if you are using cayenne pepper as a natural health remedy.

Some medications that slow blood clotting include:

• Aspirin

• Clopidogrel

* Diclofenac

* Ibuprofen

* Naproxen

* Warfarin

Capsicum can also increase how much theophylline — a bronchodilator that can treat asthma and other lung problems — the body can absorb. Therefore, taking capsicum alongside theophylline might increase the effects and side effects of theophylline.

It's wise not to use cayenne pepper on children under the age of two. It can be irritating and may lead to a negative reaction, especially on the skin.

COOKING WITH CAYENNE

Cayenne's uses in the kitchen are endless (unless you prefer a milder spice). A welcome addition to meat sauces, goulash, fish, shellfish, soup , vegetable dishes, and the spice should be used with an easy hand, and extra care.

Naturally spicy, cayenne should be simmered for hours and allowed to blend with your recipe's other ingredients before serving. The hottest parts of the pepper are located in the fruit's seeds and interior, so if you're looking for a more mild flavor, remove both before using.

If it's a fiery dish you're hungering for, by all means, use the whole pepper. If you're not sure, keep a slice of bread nearby to reduce the sting. Contrary to popular belief, a cold drink will not relieve your burning mouth. Try butter, milk, or celery instead.

If you realize the dish is too hot before serving, the spiciness can easily be lowered by adding potatoes, noodles, or coconut – along with these other cooling foods that help balance excessive spiciness.

These might just make the soup a bit more like stew, or make the chili con carne a chili-mac, but in the end it's all about making the meal enjoyable – do what you have to!

Therapeutic Properties Of Cayenne Pepper

On the medicinal side, cayenne has been experimented with for centuries, and continues to be used for its valuable therapeutic properties.

A stimulant, it aids in digestion, helps normalize blood circulation, tones the nervous system, and helps to relieve pain and inflammation.

High doses of vitamin C and beta carotene quickly convert to vitamin A when they're consumed, which is good for eye health.

Large amounts of capsaicin (an alkaloid) are also present, something that the Gale Encyclopedia of Cancer credits with reducing pain, suppressing cancer cells, and possibly even containing chemo-protective properties, documented in its use with cancer patients.

Cayenne's essential oils stimulate the skin, but when using its oils, take care not to burn yourself. Click here to read more about using essential oils in cooking. Never use cayenne oil on sensitive skin or mucous membranes.

Therapeutically, fresh or dried chilies are preferable, and far less irritating to the skin than peppers that have been cooked. Its properties as a warming spice are particularly beneficial for those suffering from arthritic joint pain.

A plaster can be used, made with three tablespoons of white flour, one teaspoon of olive oil, and one teaspoon of the ground spice.

Add enough water to create a paste, then simply cover the skin with a thin piece of cloth, spread the mixture over the cloth, and add another cloth on top (just like making a sandwich). Once you're plastered, sit back and enjoy the natural warmth, and the relief it provides your aching joints.

In essence, for those of you who like it "hot," this spicy choice not only provides a happy palate, but a happy body as well.

As with any remedy, check with your doctor before using this herb for any type of therapeutic or medicinal purpose.

Cayenne Herb Preparations

The highest amount of capsaicin is located in the lining of the seeds and the membrane from which the seeds hang. You can decrease the heat of whole cayenne by first removing the seeds.

Cayenne is a great spice for many culinary dishes. If you buy cayenne powder, buy it in small amounts because it does lose its zing fairly quickly.

Cayenne is often added in minute amounts to tincture formulas. It can warm up a formula and, because it stimulates cardiovascular function, can disperse the herbal medicine more quickly throughout the body.

It can be infused into oils and made into salves for topical treatments of aches and pains. When applying the oils and salves, be sure to take measures to avoid later touching your cayenne-infused fingers to your eyes.

Samuel Thompson used cayenne in tea blends and it is an ingredient in many composition powder recipes. Here's

Composition Powder

- Bayberry Bark (powdered) 1 ounce

- Wild Ginger ½ ounce*

- Cayenne 1 drachm

A teaspoonful of the mixture to a teacupful of boiling water is taken warm at bed-time to ward off the effects of chill, and as a general stimulant.

*We now know not to consume wild ginger because of toxicity concerns; substitute store-bought ginger

Some dosage suggestions for cayenne: Always start low and slowly increase the amount to avoid unwanted effects.

- Cayenne tea: one tsp of cayenne powder per cup of water, 2 – 4 teaspoons a day

- Cayenne tincture: 5 – 15 drops

- Cayenne pepper capsules: 2 – 4 grams a day

- Cayenne liniment: 1:8 dilution

Special Considerations

Cayenne is very irritating to the eyes. If you have contacts or if you are preparing a lot of cayenne peppers you may want to wear gloves. I've heard many stories of people burning their eyes even many hours after contact and many hand washings later.

Cayenne is commonly used in pepper spray devices. In the past five years more than 60 deaths have been attributed to law enforcement use of pepper spray in the United States.

Cayenne shouldn't be taken in large amounts during pregnancy. People on warfarin or other blood-thinning pharmaceuticals should talk to their doctor before using cayenne.

• When your peppers are dry and brittle you can take them off the string and store them in an airtight bag or container until ready to use.

• As long as they are stored in a dry, dark space, dried peppers will last for years.

These peppers were hung to dry indoors so they kept their vibrant red color. Notice teach one has a cut in them to allow for air circulation and prevent mold on the inside.

How To Make Homemade Cayenne Pepper & Pepper Flakes

And now for the easy part! Get your spice grinder or coffee grinder and make homemade cayenne pepper and pepper flakes in 10 minutes or less!

WARNING: During this process fine cayenne pepper powder will be in the air – be prepared to sneeze! When you open the lid of the grinder, keep your eyes averted until the dust settles.

Time to fill those jars and make some pepper flakes and hot pepper.

HOMEMADE HOT PEPPER FLAKES

Place dried peppers into grinder.

Grind peppers a little at a time until you reach the desired consistency. Just a couple of short pulses is all you need.

Just a couple of short pulses will give you hot pepper flakes.

HOT PEPPER POWDER

A few more pulses will give you a much finer powder – cayenne pepper.

Continue to grind to flakes to get a fine powder. Be careful of fine dust powder when you open the lid!

Storing Cayenne Pepper And Pepper Flakes

Transfer your pepper and pepper flakes into your spice jars and keep with your other herbs and spices in a dry, dark cupboard, preferably away from the heat of your oven.

Use a funnel to reduce spills.

Label and enjoy in your favorite recipes. But be warned, we find our homemade cayenne powder is much spicier than store bought powder – use small amounts, taste and adjust accordingly.

Benefits Of Cayenne Pepper For Skin, Hair And Health

In India, Cayenne pepper is not a very common ingredient in the food, but we do use it to add flavor to our food. The red, hot pepper is an amazing condiment and actually has a host of benefits for you and your body. In fact, research has indicated that because of its benefits, cayenne pepper has been used for 9000 years!

1.Treats Acne:

Cayenne is known as the 'Prince of Spices' because it contains ingredients that have amazing properties. The number one ingredient in the pepper that makes it fight against acne is the presence of 'capsaicin', an active ingredient, reduces the acne discoloration and soothes the redness of the skin. It also helps in making the dark spots disappear. Capsaicin also clears out the bad blood and cleans out the toxins which in turn prevents acne and pimples.

Things you need

• ½ a ripe avocado

• One spoon cayenne pepper

• One spoon cocoa powder

Directions:

• Mix all the three together until it becomes a smooth paste and apply on your face.

• It will work to remove the impurities from the skin and also fight bacteria.

Tip: Wash off the paste and moisturize the skin for best results.

2. Beautiful Skin

Besides Capsaicin, cayenne pepper is also rich in Vitamin C, Vitamin E, Antioxidants and Vitamin B6. All these are very good to improve the health of your skin and promote collagen production that increases the elasticity of skin. The anti-fungal and anti-allergen properties of cayenne pepper also make it a great cleanser.

Things you need

• Cayenne pepper powder

• Lemon juice

Directions

• Make a paste of the cayenne pepper powder and lemon juice and apply it lightly on your skin.

• Wash off with cool water in about 15 minutes.

Tip: Test the paste on your hand before using it on your face. Sometimes it is best to get a patch test done before applying it on your face.

3. Fights Inflammation

We mentioned before that the properties of cayenne pepper make it very good as an anti-fungal, anti-bacterial as well as an anti-inflammatory ingredient. It helps to make your skin healthy and supple.

Things you need

- 1 tbsp jojoba oil

- ½ tbsp of almond meal

- 1 tsp of cayenne pepper powder

Directions

1. Mix all the three ingredients together and make a smooth paste.

2. Put this paste on your face and let the mixture stay for half an hour.

3. Wash off with cool water.

Tip: Cayenne pepper mask may not be recommended for everyone. Your skin might not take it well. Always do a little bit of a patch test before putting the whole mask on your face.

Benefits and Uses of Cayenne Pepper for Hair

Just like it is very beneficial for your skin, cayenne pepper also has a lot of benefits for your hair. Let's check some of the best uses:

1. Shiny and Voluminous Hair

Things you need

- Cayenne pepper – freshly ground

- Honey

Directions

- Mix cayenne pepper and honey and apply it directly on your scalp.

- Now use a cellophane paper to cover your hair

- Wash it off after half an hour

Tip: Apply this paste once for at least 3-4 weeks to see a difference in your hair

2. Hair Growth

Cayenne pepper is also a great way to increase the growth of your hair. The Vitamin A that is present in Cayenne Pepper is great to repair damaged hair cells and hence helps for quick growth of hair.

Things you need

- 3 eggs

- Honey

- Cayenne pepper

- Peppermint

- Olive oil

Directions

- Stir in eggs and honey and make it into a smooth paste.

- Now add the rest of the ingredients into this mixture and use the paste on your hair roots.

• Use a cap to cover your hair and let the mask sit on your scalp for at least 40 minutes.

• Wash off with a mild, organic shampoo

Tip: You this mask at least once a month to get your hair to grow faster.

Benefits of Cayenne Pepper for Health:

By now you have seen how many benefits cayenne pepper has for your hair and skin. In fact, cayenne pepper has also great benefits for your overall health. The section below talks about all the properties of cayenne pepper that makes it such an amazing ingredient to have in your kitchen.

1. Anti-cold and flu

Cayenne pepper's most important property is the one that is imparted from capsaicin- an ingredient that makes cayenne pepper a great decongestant. Mix some lemon juice, honey and hot water and have this concoction until your cold subsides

2. Anti-Migraine

Again, the main ingredient in cayenne pepper-capsaicin is responsible for bringing relief from headache. It reduces substance 'P' that is activated during a headache and stops the neurotransmitter from sending pain signals to the brain

3. Good for digestion

Cayenne pepper stimulates the enzymes present in the digestive tract and helps to digest food much faster and easily. It is also useful when you are suffering from gas and helps relieve a gassy stomach.

4. Detoxing agent

Adding some lemon juice, a little bit of honey and cayenne pepper to a glass of warm water is a great way to detoxify your body at the beginning of your day. You should drink this every morning to help make your digestion better.

5. Prevents Blood Clots

Cayenne pepper's properties make it very effective in preventing heart attacks because these properties encourage fibrinolytic activity that helps prevent blood clots.

6. Supports Weight Loss

The best thing about cayenne pepper is that it assists in your digestion and increases metabolism so that the food gets digested better and your food regime is monitored.

7. Relieves Joint and Nerve Pain

The active ingredient in cayenne pepper is capsaicin that is a proven analgesic and often prescribed to people who have been diagnosed with arthritis. Having Cayenne pepper in your diet can help relieve these nerve and joint pains.

8. Works as Anti-Irritant

Cayenne pepper is a natural anti-irritant because of the presence of capsaicin that helps to reduce the irritants in your system.

9. Boosts Metabolism

The compound capsaicin present in cayenne pepper produces heat that boosts the metabolism in the body. This produces extra heat in the system which in turn is helpful to burn calories.

10. Reduce blood sugar levels

Cayenne pepper is a spice that helps to reduce the blood sugar levels and promotes healthy insulin levels in the body

11. Source of Vitamin A & E

The levels of Vitamin A and E are very high in cayenne pepper and this helps to keep your skin healthy. These two vitamins are also power anti-oxidants that promote a healthy body and mind

12. Treats Psoriasis

Again the compound capsaicin is essential to treat psoriasis and in many cases regular use of cayenne pepper in your diet can actually help to treat this.

13. Anti-Allergies

The best property of cayenne pepper is the fact that it is a natural anti-irritant and can suppress your allergies to a large extent.

14. Anti-Fungal Properties

Cayenne pepper not only prevent fungus from forming, but it will also destroy the pathogens that may cause fungal infections to reappear.

15. Possible Anti-Cancer Agent

Research has shown that the ingredient Capsaicin in cayenne pepper can help kill cancer cells especially that causes prostate cancer.

16. Anti-Redness Properties

Cayenne pepper is a natural anti-irritant and helps remove redness that may be caused due to any kind of allergies.

17. Helps Produce Saliva

When you include cayenne pepper in your diet, you will see that your salivary glands are functioning properly and this helps increase the production of saliva. As a result, you will have better digestion of food.

18. Promotes Longevity

All the properties of cayenne pepper also make it an excellent item that promotes longevity. Capsaicin, antioxidants and vitamins all help to increase your longevity.

19. Helps Sore Throats

Cayenne pepper, as mentioned before has anti-inflammatory properties and also is a natural analgesic. Hence it can help you in case you have a sore throat. Just add it with the tea you drink or gargle with it for instant relief

20. Anti-Bacterial Properties

The pungent flavor and aroma of cayenne pepper actually indicates that it has anti-bacterial properties and is often prescribed as a natural remedy in case of an infecrelie

21. Promotes Heart Health

Cayenne pepper is a power stimulant that helps to improve the condition of the heart and helps it to perform better. As a result your heart is in a much healthier state

22. Topical Remedy

In some cases, cayenne pepper applied topically can also help relief pain and arthritis. The only important thing you should keep in mind is that you should not have broken skin because otherwise cayenne pepper will burn a lot.

23. Remedy for Toothache

Capsaicin in cayenne pepper can help with pain relief and anti-inflammation. Just apply a lit bit of the powder on your tooth

24. Prevent Blood Pressure

Mixing cayenne pepper in a glass of warm water and drinking it opens up the blood vessels and helps blood to flow faster. As a result, it will reduce blood pressure.

25. Helps Cure Ulcers

Peptic ulcers can be easily cured with the help of cayenne pepper, make sure you add some to your daily food to prevent ulcers.

26. Improves Oral Health

When you regularly have cayenne pepper, you will be able to see that there is an increase in the salivation and as a result oral health is also promoted.

Possible Side Effects:

Too much of anything is bad and you should always have spicy food in moderation. Including too much cayenne pepper in your diet may lead to these side effects:

• Skin irritation, burning and itching

• It can also irritate the skin of the nose and the mouth

• Do not bring it near damaged skin as it might lead to severe burning

Tips, Prevention and After Care

Though cayenne pepper is safe to use by everyone, sometimes you might get severe irritation or burning, especially if your skin is broken. In such cases, wash off the affected area with cold milk or cold water to prevent the burning sensation.

Why does it work for Acne?

Cayenne Pepper in Organic Skincare Can Cure Acne

According to medical news today not only does Cayenne contain the amazing capsaicin active ingredient, but it is also rich in vitamin C, vitamin B6, vitamin E, potassium, manganese and antioxidants called flavanoids. All of these vitamins and antioxidants have numerous benefits to the skin such as vitamin C increasing collagen production and reducing acne discoloration and vitamin B6 soothing redness and fading dark spots. Capsaicin is also a counter-irritant in that it brings blood to the surface and allows the toxins to be taken away. It is anti-inflammatory and therefore soothing. It's richness in vitamins and antioxidants and its soothing anti-inflammatory, anti-fungal, anti-allergen and anti-irritant properties make Cayenne perfect for tackling acne and acne scars. And that's not all, capsaicin is also a great natural preservative, perfect for increasing the shelf-life of natural skin care products, making them effective in fighting acne longer.

LEMON, HONEY, CAYENNE CLEANSE DRINK

According to the "Master Cleanser," an updated version of the Master Cleanse detox by Stanley Burroughs, you're supposed to make a single serving of the drink with:

- 2 tablespoons fresh-squeezed lemon juice

- 2 tablespoons pure maple syrup

- 1/10 teaspoon cayenne pepper (more, to taste, if desired)

- 8 to 12 ounces of purified water

The altered version of the program uses raw honey in place of the maple syrup. It's common to make a large batch of the drink to have it on hand for when hunger strikes. Since it's the only thing you'll use for the duration of the fasting diet, you'll want to have plenty of cayenne pepper, lemon and honey available.

How to Follow the Diet

During the lemon-honey-cayenne cleanse, no solid food is allowed. All your calorie consumption comes from the drink you make with cayenne pepper, lemon and honey. You can consume the mixture whenever you're hungry, though it's recommended that you have at least six glasses every day.

Other than the Master Cleanse detox drink, dieters are advised to drink a quart of warm salt water in the morning to promote bowel movements. If dieters experience constipation, use of herbal laxative teas is permitted.

Dieters are advised to follow the diet for at least 10 days but can continue for up to 40 days if desired. There is no scientific evidence to support the recommendations. Proponents of this diet claim your body needs 10 days to eliminate toxins and the longer you stay on the program, the more weight you'll lose.

The lack of solid food sets you up for nutrient deficiencies. According to the National Academies of Sciences, Engineering, Medicine, lack of sufficient protein may lead to swelling, muscle loss and thinning hair. The Academies also says a lack of iron can lead to anemia and extreme fatigue. The effects depend on which nutrients are deficient, how deficient you are, and how long the deficiency remains.

Does the Cleanse Work?

Because of the drastic cut in caloric intake, you're likely to see some weight loss at the end of the fasting period. When you resume eating solid food, however, it's likely the weight will return quickly because the loss is not likely to be fat, but water.

A small-scale study of 84 women who used a lemon detox diet, published in the May 2015 issue of Nutrition Research, suggests that a lemon detox program reduces body fat and insulin resistance through caloric restriction. This study involved participants remaining on the fast for seven days, so there is no evidence to support the benefits over an extended period of time.

Another small-scale study featured in the March 2016 issue of the Journal of Ayurveda and Integrative Medicine involved 50 participants and looked at the short-term use of a lemon juice and honey fast. This study looked at the use of the fast for four days. The results indicate that the fast may be safe and effective in reducing fat in healthy individuals. As with the other study, there is no evidence to support participants' ability to keep the weight off in the long term.

Although these two studies show a cleansing diet has positive benefits, it's unhealthy to maintain such a restricted caloric intake for a long period of time. Doing so could have negative effects on your overall health. It's best to speak with your doctor before beginning a lemon-honey-cayenne cleanse to ensure you are healthy enough.

Cayenne Pepper Tea Benefits and Recipe.

To add some kick to your health routine, try sipping a cup of cayenne pepper tea. Typically prepared with ground cayenne pepper, fresh lemon, and purified water, this spicy brew is said to stimulate your digestive system, shield your heart health, and support weight loss.

Often used as a cooking spice, cayenne pepper is packed with a substance called capsaicin. A wealth of studies have shown that capsaicin can help reduce inflammation, a process known to play a key role in many chronic health problems. Cayenne also contains a number of antioxidants, including vitamin A and vitamin C.

While cayenne pepper tea is often consumed as part of a detox diet, many people drink the tea on a daily basis in an effort to enhance their overall health.

Benefits

At this point, there's no scientific support for the claims that cayenne pepper tea can improve your wellbeing. Despite this lack of evidence, however, proponents suggest that cayenne pepper tea offers a wide range of health benefits. These benefits include:

• Improvements in blood pressure and circulation

• Increased protection against heart disease

• Pain reduction

• Relief of cough and cold symptoms, such as sore throat

Cayenne pepper tea is also said to lift your mood and raise your energy levels, as well as promote weight loss and hair growth. When used as a detox aid, it's thought to clear toxins from your body by revving up your circulation.

The Science Behind Cayenne Pepper Tea

Many studies testing the effects of capsaicin have focused on topical use of this chemical (i.e., applying capsaicin directly to your skin, usually in the form of ointments or creams). Such studies indicate that topical use of capsaicin may soothe symptoms of conditions like osteoarthritis and low back pain.

While research on capsaicin consumption is less extensive, some preliminary studies have shown that ingesting capsaicin may help with weight loss. For instance, a small study published in the journal Clinical Nutrition in 2009 found that a combination of capsaicin and green tea helped suppress hunger in healthy volunteers.

What's more, laboratory research and tests in animals have demonstrated that consuming capsaicin could fight obesity by increasing your calorie-burning rate and promoting the breakdown of fat. There's also some preliminary evidence that following a capsaicin-rich diet may help protect against cardiovascular and metabolic issues like atherosclerosis, diabetes, and stroke.

Side Effects and Safety Concerns

Since scientists have yet to test its health effects, little is known about the safety of long-term consumption of cayenne pepper tea. However, there's some concern that cayenne pepper tea may cause gastrointestinal issues in some individuals. In addition, consuming cayenne in excessive amounts may result in liver and/or kidney damage.

Transient high blood pressure has been noted with cayenne pepper intake, particularly with higher concentrations. If you have high blood pressure or heart disease, consult your doctor before using cayenne tea.

How to Make Cayenne Pepper Tea

Fans of cayenne pepper tea often prepare the brew by stirring ¼ teaspoon of ground cayenne pepper into a cup of hot water. Squeezing in the juice from half of a fresh lemon can improve the taste of your cayenne pepper tea.

When preparing your cayenne pepper tea, bring the water nearly to a boil and immediately combine with the ground cayenne pepper. For best results, stir the mixture until the cayenne has completely dissolved. You can also promote steeping by covering the mug for several minutes prior to sipping.

To add more flavor to your cayenne pepper tea—and possibly boost its health benefits—consider including other herbs in the brew. Try pepping up your tea with ingredients like ginger and turmeric, two herbs known to possess anti-inflammatory properties.

For further flavor enhancement, try stirring a teaspoon of honey into your cayenne pepper tea.

A word of advice: cayenne pepper tea often causes a burning sensation at the back of the throat, but sipping slowly may help alleviate that burning and—in turn—greatly increase your enjoyment of your tea.

Cayenne, Ginger, & Lemon Shot

This is a classic juice shot. It's great for when you're feeling under the weather or partied a little too hard the night before. This shot cleanses the body, detoxifies the organs, and boosts metabolism. What more could you ask for?

You get all the aforementioned benefits of cayenne, plus all of the good ginger and lemon have to offer. Ginger is powerful antioxidant and antiinflammatory. It soothes upset stomachs and aids digestion, like cayenne. It also boosts your immune system and fights infection, since it is naturally antimicrobial. Ginger also stimulates your metabolism and allows you to burn more calories and fat, similarly to cayenne. It can even help your body recover faster and more efficiently after a hard workout, thanks to its antiinflammatory properties. Plus, ginger helps to regulate blood sugar and helps fight cravings. Lemon works wonders for your immune system, due to its high content of Vitamin C. It helps to alkalinize the body, thus keeping the body balanced and healthy. Lemon also boasts lots of detoxifying antioxidants. This cayenne, ginger, and lemon shot is a great way to start your day.

Ingredients:

• Juice of ½ a lemon

• 1 large knob of ginger

• Pinch of cayenne pepper

Peel your ginger and add it to your juicer or blender. Mix the ginger juice with the lemon juice and add the cayenne. Stir well. Then down the hatch! Cheers!

Ginger Turmeric Wellness Shot Recipe

Ginger turmeric shots with lemon, cayenne, and orange. These wellness shots have powerful anti-inflammatory and immune boosting properties!

When we think of shots, "healthy" is usually the last thing that comes to mind.

But wellness shots are a recent health trend that's really taking over. These potent little tonics pack a concentrated dose of vitamins, micronutrients, and antioxidants.

They're being used for everything from an energy boost, to gut health, and even to fight inflammation depending on the ingredients you use!

Wellness or "booster" shots are a common addition to juice cleanses as a little something extra in between the main juices. They're on my list of recommendations for juice cleanse beginners because they can help to boost your energy during a cleanse.

But these ginger turmeric shots are specifically made for their anti-inflammatory properties. They're also great for boosting our immune systems.

Not to mention they taste like little bottles of sunshine (trust me that's a real flavor).

Turmeric Ginger Shot Benefits

So what makes these wellness shots so healthy?

The main active ingredients are gingerols (from ginger) and curcumin (from turmeric). These plant compounds have powerful medicinal properties with a variety of potential health benefits.

• ANTI-INFLAMMATORY PROPERTIES

Recent studies have found that chronic inflammation is linked to many major modern diseases, including heart disease and cancer.

The curcumin found in turmeric has been shown to have extremely powerful anti-inflammatory effects. Curcumin has actually been shown to be as effective at treating inflammation as some modern prescription drugs.

Ginger is also known for its anti-inflammatory properties. One study found ginger extract helped to significantly reduce pain in patients with osteoarthritis.

• FIGHTS INFECTION

Gingerol is a very effective anti-bacterial compound, helping to fight infection by preventing the growth of harmful pathogens.

Turmeric also has immune supporting properties. Curcumin is able to modulate the immune response and even enhance antibody responses, improving our bodies natural defense systems.

BUT WHY SHOTS?

Through juicing, we are able to get a very concentrated dose of gingerol and curcumin that would be difficult to achieve any other way.

Turmeric and ginger are both known for the "spicy" burning sensation they have when eaten. That's why shots are the perfect method of delivery for this healthy juice.

A glass full of straight ginger or turmeric juice would be pretty unpleasant, but shots mixed with added lemon and orange juice are delicious!

The strong flavors of turmeric and ginger also make them great for flavoring other healthy juices without the need to add lots of high sugar fruits.

HOW TO MAKE GINGER TURMERIC SHOTS

1. PREP INGREDIENTS

Wash and dry the fresh produce. Peel the lemons and oranges. Cut the fresh produce to size so that it will fit in your juicer.

2. BOIL TURMERIC

Bring ¾ cup of water to a boil in a small pan. Once the water is boiling, add about ¼ cup of turmeric root and boil it for 10 minutes.

After 10 minutes, remove the turmeric root while reserving the liquid in the pan. Put liquid in the fridge to cool.

 Fresh Tip: Heating the turmeric first helps to increase the absorption of its main active ingredient – curcumin.

3. ADD TO JUICER

Using a juicer, juice the turmeric root, ginger root, lemons, and oranges.

Stir in the cayenne pepper, black pepper. Stir in the remaining cooled liquid from boiling the turmeric.

*Optional: To help with absorption, stir in ¼ tsp of oil if you aren't taking the shots with food.

HOW TO INCREASE ABSORPTION OF TURMERIC SHOTS

The curcumin in turmeric is a powerful anti-inflammatory compound, but unfortunately it is poorly absorbed by our bodies.

Luckily, there are a few ways we can substantially increase curcumin's effectiveness and absorption rate.

Black Pepper: Black pepper contains a compound called "piperine" which has been shown to increase absorption of curcumin by up to 2000%!

Heat: Studies found that heating turmeric first can help to increase the absorption of curcumin without degrading it.

Fat: Curcumin is fat soluble. To get the most out of turmeric shots it's important to add a small amount of fat like an oil or take them with a meal that has fat in it.

WILL TURMERIC POWDER WORK INSTEAD OF FRESH TURMERIC?

Sometimes fresh turmeric root can be hard to find at local supermarkets.

You can replace the turmeric root in this recipe with about 2 tbsp of turmeric powder or 4 servings of turmeric powder supplements.

If you go this route, I recommend a turmeric powder extract, not just any old turmeric from the spice shelf.

Turmeric on the spice shelf may only be 3% curcumin by weight where as extracts can be up to 95% curcumin!

If you don't have a juicer (or don't want your hands stained orange for the day), you can still try these potent little health tonics at most cold pressed juice bars.

Ginger turmeric shots 2

Ginger turmeric shots with lemon, cayenne, and orange. These wellness shots have powerful anti-inflammatory and immune boosting properties!

INGREDIENTS

• 4 inches Turmeric Root (about ¼ cup fresh or 2 tbsp powder)

• 4 inches Ginger Root (about ¼ cup)

• 2 Lemons, peeled

• 2 Oranges, peeled

• ¾ cup Water

• 1/8 tsp Cayenne Pepper

• 1/8 tsp ground Black Pepper (for turmeric absorption)

• ¼ tsp Oil.

INSTRUCTIONS

• Wash and dry fresh produce. Peel the lemons and oranges.

• Bring ¾ cup of water to a boil in a small pan. Once boiling, add turmeric root, reduce heat to medium high and simmer for 7-8 minutes. After simmering, remove turmeric root while reserving the liquid in the pan. Put liquid in fridge to cool.

• While liquid cools, juice the turmeric root, ginger root, lemons, and oranges in a juicer. Stir in the cayenne, black pepper, and oil. Stir in the remaining cooled liquid from boiling the turmeric.

• Pour into shot glasses and enjoy! Store the leftover ginger turmeric shots in an air tight container in the fridge. They will last about 2-3 days.

NOTES

The active ingredient in turmeric called "curcumin" is not easily absorbed by our bodies. A compound called "piperine" in black pepper increases the absorption of curcumin by 2000%.

Absorption is also increased by heating the turmeric. Curcumin is fat soluble so adding oil or taking the shots with a meal will increase their effectiveness.

NUTRITION

Serving Size: 1 shot Calories: 21 Sugar: 7g Sodium: 3mg Fat: 0g Saturated Fat: 0g Unsaturated Fat: 0g Trans Fat: 0g Carbohydrates: 10g Fiber: 0g Protein: 0g Cholesterol: 0g

CONCLUSION

Cayenne is a shrub that grows long pods called chili peppers. The pepper's active ingredient, capsaicin, is valued for its therapeutic effects.

Cayenne pepper is consumed in whole and powder forms for its health benefits. You'll find capsaicin supplements or topical creams online or in health food stores.

Some of the most well-known cayenne pepper benefits include its ability to aid digestion, relieve migraines, prevent blood clots, promote detoxification, relieve pain, support weight loss and boost metabolism.